Clinical Governance in Gastroenterology

Key points for primary care

Greg Rubin

Roger Jones

Jim Price

and

Richard Stevens

The Primary Care Society for

D1333477

RADCLIFFE MEDICAL PRESS

Radcliffe Medical Press Ltd
18 Marcham Road, Abingdon, Oxon OX14 1AA

British Library Cataloguing in Publication Data

A catalogue record for this book is available from the British Library.

ISBN 1 85775 438 7

Typeset by Joshua Associates Ltd, Oxford
Printed and bound by TJ International Ltd, Padstow, Cornwall

Contents

About the authors

Greg Rubin FRCGP is Professor of Primary Care at the University of Sunderland and Secretary of the Primary Care Society for Gastroenterology. He is a practising GP with a long-standing research interest in the management of gastrointestinal problems in primary care and at the primary–secondary care interface.

Roger Jones MA DM FRCP FRCGP FFPHM FMEdSci is Wolfson Professor of General Practice at Guy's, King's and St Thomas' School of Medicine London, Chairman of the European Society for Primary Care Gastroenterology, President of the Primary Care Society for Gastroenterology in the UK and Editor of *Family Practice*. He has been involved in research into the epidemiology, natural history and management of gastrointestinal disorders in general practice for 20 years.

Jim Price MA MRCP(UK) MRCGP is a full-time GP in Chichester, West Sussex and Vice Chairman and Clinical Governance Lead for the Chichester & Rural PCG. He is a Committee member of the Primary Care Society for Gastroenterology and a Board member of Medical Managers in Primary Care. His interests include quality, leadership, education and management in primary care, and his recent research has been concerned with perceptions of quality in endoscopy services. He continues to offer a flexible sigmoidoscopy service in his practice.

Richard Stevens MA FRCGP is Chairman of the Primary Care Society for Gastroenterology. He is a practising GP in Oxford and an endoscopist at the John Radcliffe Hospital. He is attached to the Department of Primary Health Care at the University of Oxford.

Chapter 1

Introduction

The establishment of primary care groups (PCGs) and primary care trusts (PCTs) offers an exciting opportunity to provide coherent primary care services for defined populations, and also to integrate these services, as far as possible, with social care, housing and education on the one hand and with secondary care on the other. However, PCG/PCT Chairs and clinical governance leads face considerable challenges in determining the best ways to configure and commission services, particularly in relation to the emerging National Service Frameworks and the demands of clinical governance and evidence-based medicine.

The Primary Care Society for Gastroenterology (PCSG) was set up 15 years ago to provide a focus for general practitioners with research and clinical interests in gastroenterology, and to promote high standards in the clinical care of patients with gastrointestinal problems. Recognising both the opportunities and the challenges presented by new structures in the NHS, the PCSG has produced this short book, *Clinical Governance in Gastroenterology*, to help

PCGs/PCTs, health authorities and secondary care specialists to understand and respond to the burden of illness and the requirements of care of patients with gastrointestinal disorders.

In this book, we have identified 17 key topics and systematically examined each of them in a way which we hope will be helpful to the reader. We have introduced each topic with a definition of the subject under consideration and then explained the significance of the problem, particularly in terms of the numbers of patients or procedures likely to be encountered within a notional PCG/PCT with a population of 100 000. We have then listed key clinical points (related to presentation, investigation and diagnosis) and key therapeutic points (related to the use of medication, surgery and other therapeutic interventions). We have pointed out where to find guidelines (regional, national and international) if these exist, and also where to find information for patients, with details of useful websites. We have included a section on access to services, indicating which hospital-based investigations or other services are required for effective management of the condition. The section on risk management gives examples of ways in which individual practices, or groups of practices, can review clinical activity (diagnosis, prescribing and referral) and use techniques such as audit and critical incident analysis to draw conclusions about effective management. Each chapter contains a section on health economics, in which we have attempted to highlight the most prominent areas of resource utilisation related to each topic under consideration. Finally, we have included notes on data management, as we believe that accurate record-keeping and data entry are prerequisites not only for audit but also for effective clinical care.

As far as possible the information contained in this book is based on the research evidence, and is drawn from a wide range of source documents. The essential resource for detailed patient information on each of the subjects covered is the Digestive Disorders Foundation website at www.digestivedisorders.org.uk. An extensive UK-oriented source of links to patient groups, fact sheets, publications and research can be found at www.patient.co.uk. Finally, we acknowledge the invaluable source material in texts edited by Bodger *et al.* and by McDonald *et al.*

This book offers a template for clinical governance, supporting and informing those responsible for the delivery of high-quality care in gastroenterology. However, we also hope that it will be a responsive and flexible tool for its users, incorporating new evidence as it becomes available and responding to comments and suggestions. To this end, an important medium for future publication will be the World Wide Web. The text will be placed on the website of the Primary Care Society for Gastroenterology, www.pcsg.org.uk, and will be regularly revised. It will also be available at www.primarycareonline.co.uk. We invite and welcome feedback via the PCSG Secretariat, and will incorporate your responses at each revision.

Further reading

Bodger K, Daly M and Heatley RV (eds) (2000) *Clinical Economics in Gastroenterology.* Blackwell Science, Oxford.
McDonald J, Burroughs A and Feagan B (eds) (1999) *Evidence-Based Gastroenterology and Hepatology.* BMJ Books, London.

Contact details

PCSG Secretariat, Department of Primary Health Care, Institute of Health Sciences, Old Road, Headington, Oxford OX3 7LF.

Chapter 2

The structures of clinical governance

Within healthcare in the UK, a veritable blizzard of rhetoric and legislation has overtaken the issue of quality in practice, reinventing it as clinical governance. However, peer-led organisations and structures to maintain and promote good-quality practice within the health professions are not new. Indeed, concern for quality and standards could be claimed to be a defining feature of a 'profession'. In recent times, two important changes have moved these issues much closer to centre stage, and have driven demands for greater public accountability. There has been political and public concern about high-profile examples of poor clinical performance, of which the events in Bristol are a much-quoted example. There has also been a growing public and professional awareness that healthcare resources are limited, and that some means of achieving equitable access for patients to effective and cost-effective treatments is necessary.

Clinical governance is seen as a framework which draws together the different activities that constitute quality improvement. Ten processes that constitute clinical governance were identified in the white paper, *The New NHS: modern, dependable*, together with two new organisations to ensure that they were implemented.

The processes of clinical governance

These are as follows:

- evidence-based practice and the infrastructure to support it

- systematic dissemination of good practice, ideas and innovation

- quality improvement processes such as clinical audit

- high-quality data to monitor clinical care

- clinical risk reduction programmes

- adverse events detected and openly investigated, and the lessons learned promptly applied

- lessons for clinical practice systematically learned from complaints made by patients

- problems of poor clinical performance recognised at an early stage and dealt with appropriately

- all professional development programmes to reflect principles of clinical governance

- leadership skills development at the clinical team level.

Two key organisations underpin the processes of clinical governance. The National Institute for Clinical Excellence (NICE) will provide national service frameworks (guidelines, algorithms, protocols) which will be audited by the Commission for Health Improvement (CHI) according to a series of agreed parameters (minimum datasets).

National Institute for Clinical Excellence

NICE is constituted as a special health authority with 'such functions in connection with the promotion of clinical excellence as the Secretary of State may direct'. Put simply, it is concerned with the effectiveness and affordability of healthcare interventions. There is therefore an explicit acknowledgement that NICE will provide the criteria for some form of rationing process, under Government direction. On the other hand, it may prove an important means of promoting equity of access, notably to expensive therapies. Key to its functions is the Appraisals Committee, the function of which is to consider evidence on new or established health technologies and to provide advice to the Board.

Much of the lay publicity surrounding NICE has concerned its evaluation of new technologies, notably sildenafil and beta-interferon. However, it is also producing a raft of guidance documents on the processes of clinical care, such as referral, which will have a much greater impact on clinical practice. There is still uncertainty about the capacity of NICE to keep pace with the emergence of new technologies and at the same time to consider the effectiveness of existing practices and therapies.

Commission for Health Improvement

The enforcing arm of this new quality assurance system is the Commission for Health Improvement (CHI), which will ensure that health service organisations systematically and consistently take account of NICE's guidelines. However, the Prime Minister's own description is of a standards watchdog that will 'go round every hospital and PCG/PCT in the country rooting out bad practice and ensuring that the best treatments, as recommended by NICE, are being used'. As such, the early concept of CHI as a source of constructive criticism and advice appears to have been lost.

In practice, it seems likely that CHI will start its work with pilot studies of a spread of acute trusts, and then PCGs, in order to test a possible review methodology. This may well be based on that used by the Audit Commission. In other words, it will be risk based and will initially rely on organisations to demonstrate their competence in self-regulation. In all this there is a danger of over-monitoring, to the detriment of healthcare provision, and sensitivity to the balance of costs and benefits will be important.

Chapter 3

Investigations

Many patients with gastrointestinal problems can usefully be investigated in the primary care setting, where investigations are likely to be used either to make a diagnosis or to provide information in anticipation of a hospital out-patient visit. The investigations listed below include those to which general practitioners should reasonably expect to have direct access.

Upper gastrointestinal endoscopy

This is likely to be the first-line investigation for patients with unexplained, persistent upper gastrointestinal symptoms that require investigation (*see* Chapter 4 on dyspepsia and Chapter 5 on gastro-oesophageal reflux disease). The procedure has a much higher sensitivity and specificity for identification of mucosal lesions than radiological studies, it enables biopsies (of suspicious lesions and to test for *Helicobacter pylori* infection) to be taken, and it is often better tolerated by elderly, relatively immobile subjects than a barium meal. The risk of cardiorespiratory depression needs to be considered if sedated endoscopy is planned in patients with compromised cardiac or pulmonary function, although most upper gastrointestinal endoscopies are now performed without sedation, using only an anaesthetic throat spray. The procedure has implications for patients' ability to return home from hospital alone (inadvisable) and to drive or operate machinery the following day (also ill-advised when sedation is used).

Barium meal examinations

These are much less frequently used when gastro-oesophageal reflux disease or ulcer disease is suspected, because of the superior accuracy of upper gastrointestinal endoscopy. However, a well-conducted double-contrast barium meal can still show detailed gastroduodenal anatomy, and may be useful for defining the anatomy when, for example, gastric outflow problems are suspected or an epigastric mass is found for which the cause is uncertain. Barium studies are not particularly helpful for making the diagnosis of gastro-oesophageal reflux, although oesophageal ulcers can be detected and the extent of hiatal herniation assessed.

Barium swallow examinations

These are useful in patients with disorders of swallowing, particularly when motility disorders of the oesophagus (e.g. achalasia or stricture) are suspected. A 'marshmallow swallow' may be helpful for delineating the extent of oesophageal dysmotility.

Oesophageal manometry and pH monitoring

These investigations are rarely available on a direct-access basis, and are generally employed when the diagnosis of gastro-oesophageal reflux disease or an oesophageal motility disorder is either suspected or equivocal. Their interpretation can be problematic, and the decision to undertake these investigations is generally best left to a gastroenterologist.

Barium enema examinations

These remain useful for investigating patients with lower bowel problems. A well-conducted double-contrast barium enema, in which the colon is visualised as far as the caecum, can provide valuable information about mucosal abnormalities (e.g. in inflammatory bowel disease) and anatomical distortion (e.g. tumour, diverticulitis), and may, depending on local expertise, provide a more accurate assessment of the colon than a less well-performed colonoscopy. Patients often find barium enemas unpleasant, and old people may find the pre-radiology bowel preparation taxing.

Flexible sigmoidoscopy

This is the early investigation of choice for unexplained rectal bleeding. It is often used in conjunction with a double-contrast barium enema, and is likely to emerge as a screening modality for colorectal cancer. The timely investigation of patients with suspicious lower bowel symptoms, particularly rectal bleeding, is crucially dependent on general practitioners and specialists working closely together to provide a 'fast-track service' for patients in whom malignancy is suspected. Flexible sigmoidoscopy is an important part of the pathway of investigation.

Colonoscopy

This is undertaken when it is necessary to inspect the entire colon, either as a diagnostic procedure or as part of surveillance in patients with long-standing inflammatory bowel disease, polyps, etc. The procedure is performed under sedation and is not without risk (e.g. of perforation and haemorrhage). A well-conducted colonoscopy has excellent sensitivity and specificity for the identification of mucosal lesions, but the procedure is highly operator-dependent, with some units failing to reach the caecum in up to 25% of examinations, a rate which is barely acceptable.

Haematological investigations

These may be helpful in patients with suspected gastrointestinal lesions causing blood loss (haemoglobin, film, ferritin), or in patients in whom inflammatory bowel disease or malignancy are suspected (erythrocyte sedimentation rate (ESR), although this investigation has poor sensitivity and specificity for inflammatory bowel disease).

Biochemical investigations

These are frequently used in patients with hepatobiliary disorders. Liver function tests (gamma-glutamyl transpeptidase (GGT), alanine aminotransferase (ALT) and aspartate aminotransferase (AST)) are important in diagnosing and monitoring hepatitis, cholestasis and obstructive conditions, while a full range of microbiological investigations is needed for the evaluation of hepatitis in general practice (hepatitis A, B and C antigens, Epstein–Barr virus and cytomegalovirus). A random amylase estimation may be useful in patients with recurrent, undiagnosed upper abdominal pain.

Helicobacter pylori *testing*

This can be undertaken in a variety of ways. At present, surgery-based near-patient tests for *Helicobacter pylori* are not recommended because of their inferior sensitivity and specificity compared to ELISA investigations performed in the hospital laboratory, although more accurate test kits are under development. For the time being, general practitioners should use a hospital-based ELISA test for *Helicobacter pylori* antibodies, to determine the presence of infection, and a C_{13} or C_{14} urea breath test (UBT) to check for eradication of *Helicobacter*. Once again, hospital-based UBTs are recommended unless a very large practice is undertaking large numbers of these tests.

Endomysial antibodies

These are a sensitive and specific test for coeliac disease. Recent primary care research has indicated that this condition is more common than was previously suspected, and in patients with suspicious features an endomysial antibody (EMA) test should be ordered.

Lactose intolerance

Although rarely considered in the differential diagnosis of irritable bowel syndrome (IBS), lactose intolerance is occasionally responsible for functional bowel symptoms. A xylose absorption test should be considered in patients with unexplained lower bowel symptoms which do not fit the clinical picture of IBS.

Guidelines

See Chapter 4 on dyspepsia and Chapter 5 on gastro-oesophageal reflux disease for guidelines on the use of endoscopy in the investigation of dyspepsia and gastro-oesophageal reflux symptoms.

Access to services

The majority of the investigations listed above should be available on a direct-access basis for general practitioners, and if they are not, the PCG/PCT should attempt to secure access. A direct-access endoscopy service with a waiting-list of much over 4–6 weeks is unacceptable, so the waiting time for investigations and the speed and format of reporting (which should always include a clear statement not only of diagnosis and management but also of the responsibility – hospital or GP – for follow-up) should also be included in a service-level agreement.

Risk management

- In upper gastrointestinal disorders, patients with gastric cancer can usefully form critical incident cases for review of the use of upper gastrointestinal investigations.

- Patients with inflammatory bowel disease are often useful cases to use as critical incidents, for examining delays in diagnosis and the use of investigations.

- Any patient with colorectal cancer represents a useful opportunity for a critical incident discussion of the availability and use of investigations and management.

Health economics

The cost of these investigations varies considerably, and indicative costs have not been included here because they are likely to become outdated or inapplicable to individual trusts. However, many of these investigations are relatively expensive and should therefore be used judiciously.

Chapter 4

Dyspepsia

Introduction

Dyspepsia can be defined as upper abdominal or retrosternal pain or discomfort, generally related to the presence of food, and sometimes accompanied by other digestive symptoms, including heartburn, epigastric burning, early satiety and (less commonly) abdominal bloating and generalised discomfort. There are three types of dyspepsia, namely reflux-like, ulcer-like and dysmotility-like, although there is considerable overlap between these, and the clinical symptoms are often a poor guide to their origin.

Significance

Dyspepsia is a common problem in the community, affecting up to 40% of individuals in any one year. It accounts for 4–5% of consultations in primary care, and can be the presenting symptom of a number of serious conditions, including oesophageal and gastric cancer and peptic ulceration. Up to 60% of patients who present with dyspepsia in general practice do not have a readily identifiable organic cause for their problems on investigation. This is known as functional dyspepsia, which may prove to be a long-standing and troublesome problem.

Key clinical points

- Only about 25% of patients consult, and concerns about the meaning and possible seriousness of symptoms are important reasons for consultation.

- Alarm symptoms include difficulty or pain on swallowing, weight loss, persistent pain despite therapy, evidence of bleeding and new dyspeptic symptoms in patients aged 50 years or over. Any of these should prompt early investigation, preferably by endoscopy.

- Routine testing for *Helicobacter pylori* in all dyspeptic patients is not recommended, but may be useful prior to making a decision about further investigations, including endoscopy.

- A clear explanation of the condition and the identification of aggravating lifestyle factors are as important as investigation and drug therapy.

- In patients with long-term, relapsing symptoms, a 'once-in-a-lifetime' endoscopy may be appropriate to exclude an organic cause.

Key therapeutic points

- When peptic ulcer disease and reflux oesophagitis have been excluded, the therapeutic choice is between acid-suppressing drugs, namely H_2-receptor antagonists or proton pump inhibitors, and the use of prokinetic agents.

- Long-term treatment of functional (non-organic) dyspepsia without adequate investigation is not recommended.

Guidelines

British Society of Gastroenterology (1996) *Dyspepsia Management Guidelines.* British Society of Gastroenterology, London.
Primary Care Society for Gastroenterology (1999) *Decision Points in the Management of* H. pylori *in Primary Care.* Primary Care Society for Gastroenterology, Oxford; www.pcsg.org.uk

Access to services

Ready access to upper gastrointestinal endoscopy is important. Around 1–2% of the general adult population may be expected to require an endoscopy each year.

Long waiting times for gastroscopy may result in patients being prescribed acid-suppressing drugs as an interim measure. There is evidence that gastric cancer is more likely to be missed at endoscopy if a course of proton pump inhibitors has been taken prior to the procedure.

Carbon urea breath tests or hospital laboratory serology testing are recommended for diagnosis of *Helicobacter pylori* infection. Near-patient serology tests are not sufficiently sensitive or specific for this purpose. The urea breath test (which is also prescribable on FP10) is recommended for confirming eradication of *Helicobacter pylori.*

Risk management

Suitable topics for risk management include the following:

- significant event analysis of patients with a new diagnosis of upper gastrointestinal cancer

- significant event analysis of patients who develop serious complications of peptic ulcer disease

- review of patients on long-term acid suppression therapy (with H_2-blockers and proton pump inhibitors) to identify those who require further investigation

- patients with peptic ulcer disease who have not yet received *Helicobacter pylori* eradication should be considered for eradication therapy

- patients who have previously been given eradication therapy and who are now back on acid-suppression therapy should have their diagnosis and management reviewed.

Health economics

Dyspepsia represents a considerable burden in terms of prescribing and investigations, which should be minimised in patients without alarm symptoms. Local provision of endoscopy, based in primary care, may be considered in order to reduce the cost of investigations, and long-term treatment with acid-suppressing drugs requires periodic scrutiny. On the basis of predictive modelling, a *Helicobacter pylori* 'test and treat' strategy for dyspepsia is likely to be a cheaper option than initial endoscopy, although evidence with regard to clinical effectiveness and long-term benefit is currently lacking.

Chapter 5

Gastro-oesophageal reflux disease

Introduction

Gastro-oesophageal reflux disease (GORD) is an increasingly common problem in the community, in general practice and in secondary care. In GORD, lower oesophageal sphincter dysfunction allows gastric acid (and sometimes bile) to reflux into the oesophagus, causing characteristic symptoms and oesophageal damage. It is important to appreciate that GORD may be either endoscopy-negative (when the typical symptoms of heartburn are caused by oesophageal acid exposure without oesophagitis) or endoscopy-positive (when a range of oesophageal lesions, from erythema to circumferential ulceration, stricture and haemorrhage, may be present – this is known as reflux oesophagitis). Reflux oesophagitis was originally classified according to the Savary–Miller criteria, but the new Los Angeles system of classification is now being used to characterise the endoscopic changes seen in patients with GORD.

GORD is a chronic and relapsing condition. Long-standing GORD is associated with the development of intestinal metaplasia in the oesophagus (Barrett's oesophagus), which in turn is a precursor of oesophageal adenocarcinoma.

Significance

Symptoms suggestive of GORD are common in the community, perhaps affecting 30% of people each year, but not all of these individuals have GORD. Many of them will have intermittent, mild reflux symptoms which should be regarded as normal. Patients with GORD have more persistent, chronic symptoms, although their presentation may not always be typical, and atypical chest pain can present diagnostic problems. Because GORD is a long-term, relapsing condition, for which acid suppression is the most effective therapy, the costs of treatment can be substantial. If the symptoms of GORD are severe or complications such as stricture formation occur, the impact on the patient's quality of life is considerable. It appears that the population prevalence and rate of diagnosis of GORD in Western and other cultures are both gradually increasing.

Key clinical points

- In patients with typical reflux symptoms (heartburn and retro-sternal burning, with or without acid regurgitation), a reasonably secure clinical diagnosis of GORD can be made as the basis for initial therapy.

- If reflux symptoms begin in patients over the age of 50 years, or are accompanied by alarm symptoms including pain and difficulty on swallowing, urgent endoscopic investigation is mandatory.

- If symptoms are atypical or difficult to interpret, relatively early endoscopy may be required to settle the issue. An alternative which has yet to be evaluated fully is the acid-suppression test, in which the symptomatic response to a double dose of proton pump inhibitors given for 1 to 2 weeks is used as a test for GORD.

- There is mounting support for the concept of a 'once-in-a-lifetime' endoscopy to make a firm diagnosis and to exclude patients with Barrett's oesophagus or overt malignancy.

- There are arguments both for and against endoscopic surveillance of Barrett's oesophagus. In the absence of a definitive study it is difficult to disregard current recommendations for surveillance endoscopy every 1–2 years until evidence to the contrary is available.

- Further investigation of patients with reflux symptoms is sometimes required. pHmetry is a difficult and inconsistent investigation, and oesophageal manometry is only available in specialist centres.

Key therapeutic points

- Therapy for GORD should be symptom led rather than endoscopy driven. The exceptions to this are severe oesophagitis and Barrett's oesophagus, when continuous maintenance therapy is necessary.

- There is still controversy over whether a 'step-up' approach (in which therapy is gradually increased to achieve symptom control) or a 'step-down' approach (in which treatment starts with relatively high-dose therapy, tapering the dosage to the level at which symptoms are controlled) is preferable. The cost-effectiveness of these approaches is still being evaluated.

- Control of symptoms with the lowest effective dose of acid-suppressing agent, usually a proton pump inhibitor, should be the goal, and although daily maintenance therapy may be recommended, patients are more likely to take their medication in response to symptoms.

- Intermittent or on-demand treatment with a proton pump inhibitor is effective in managing symptoms of heartburn in half of all patients with uncomplicated GORD.

- Surgery for GORD (open or laparoscopic fundoplication) has a place in the management of this disease, although the procedure has a significant morbidity and a small but definite mortality. Patient selection, generally of younger patients facing very long-term drug therapy, should be discussed carefully with specialist colleagues.

- Other therapeutic modalities, including prokinetic agents, have a relatively small part to play in the management of GORD. In refractory patients, cotherapy with a proton pump inhibitor may be useful.

- There is no evidence that eradication of *Helicobacter pylori* contributes to the effective management of GORD.

Guidelines

Kroes RM *et al.* (1999) Gastro-oesophageal reflux disease in primary care. *Eur J Gen Pract.* **5**: 88–97.

Dent J *et al.* (1999) An evidence-based appraisal of reflux disease management; the Genval Workshop Report. *Gut.* **44** (Supplement 2); http://gut.bmjjournals.com/content/vol44/suppl_2/

Access to services

Timely access to upper gastrointestinal endoscopy is likely to be helpful for managing some patients with GORD, particularly older patients and those with atypical symptoms. Oesophageal manometry and pHmetry are second-line investigations, and selection of patients for these procedures is best left to specialists.

Risk management

- Repeat prescribing for proton pump inhibitors is a suitable topic for practice prescribing audit.

- Patients who develop complications of GORD or Barrett's oesophagus/oesophageal cancer can form the basis of a critical incident analysis.

Health economics

Proton pump inhibitors are extensively used for the treatment of GORD, and the cost of their prescription in the community was £291 million in 1998 – over half a million pounds per PCG/PCT. Appropriate rates and levels of prescribing (half-dose proton pump inhibitors are often adequate to maintain symptom control in GORD) need to be examined carefully. On-demand therapy is now emerging as an acceptable and cost-effective modality, at least in patients with endoscopy-negative or Los Angeles A and B oesophagitis.

Chapter 6

Peptic ulcer disease

Introduction

Peptic ulceration is a non-neoplastic break in the mucosa of the stomach or duodenum that extends through the muscularis mucosae. *Helicobacter pylori* infection, smoking and use of non-steroidal anti-inflammatory drugs (NSAIDs) are the three major environmental risk factors, together with intrinsic factors such as genetic predisposition and acid hypersecretion. The peak ages of onset of peptic ulcer disease (PUD) are 20–40 years for duodenal ulcer and 50–70 years for gastric ulcer. Prior to the advent of *H. pylori* eradication therapies, PUD was a chronic relapsing disorder.

Significance

PUD is responsible for 4500 deaths each year in the UK. Its annual incidence rate is about 200 per 100 000 per year, 85% of which are duodenal ulcers. Peptic ulceration is the diagnosis in 10–15% of open-access gastroscopies. The point prevalence of active peptic ulcer is 1–2%.

The advent of effective regimes for the eradication of *H. pylori* allows the cure of PUD. Patients in whom eradication is successful experience relapse rates of 4–5% per annum, compared to 54–67% in those who remain infected.

Key clinical points

- PUD cannot be reliably distinguished from other causes of dyspepsia on the basis of symptoms alone.

- *H. pylori* infection is present in 95% of patients with duodenal ulcer and in 70% of those with gastric ulcer.

- Although about 30% of the general population are infected with *H. pylori*, PUD is present in only 14% of patients with dyspepsia who present to their GP.

- Gastroscopy is the most appropriate investigation if PUD is suspected. It allows direct inspection of the mucosa as well as biopsy for histology and diagnosis of *H. pylori* infection. Haematological tests are of limited value.

- Carbon urea breath tests or laboratory ELISA serology are the most suitable non-invasive tests for the diagnosis of *H. pylori* infection. Near-patient tests are insufficiently sensitive, and in one study it was found that they would have missed one-third of all peptic ulcers.

- The restriction of gastroscopy to patients who test positive for *H. pylori* results in a 30% reduction in procedures (test and endoscope strategy).

Key therapeutic points

- The primary treatment for PUD is the eradication of *H. pylori* infection. The currently recommended regime is a standard dose of a proton pump inhibitor, amoxicillin 1000 mg and clarithromycin 500 mg, all administered twice daily for 7 days.

- Treatment failures should receive a proton pump inhibitor twice daily together with bismuth triple therapy (colloidal bismuth substitute 240 mg, metronidazole 400 mg, tetracycline 500 mg, all four times daily) for 7–14 days.

- *H. pylori* testing to confirm eradication is unnecessary in uncomplicated duodenal ulcer disease. Patients with gastric ulcer should have healing of the ulcer and eradication of *H. pylori* confirmed by gastroscopy.

- Patients with complicated PUD should remain on acid-suppressing therapy until *H. pylori* eradication has been confirmed.

Guidelines

British Society of Gastroenterology (1996) *Dyspepsia Management Guidelines*. British Society of Gastroenterology, London.
Primary Care Society for Gastroenterology (1999) *Decision Points in the Management of* H. pylori *in Primary Care*. Primary Care Society for Gastroenterology, Oxford; www.pcsg.org.uk

Access to services

See Chapter 4 on dyspepsia.

Risk management

- Patients previously shown to have PUD and who are symptomatic or on long-term acid-suppression therapy should be offered *H. pylori* eradication therapy.

- An evidence-based approach to *H. pylori* eradication should include protocols which address the use of *H. pylori* testing and gastroscopy in the management of dyspepsia.

Health economics

Theoretical cost-effectiveness analyses show that for patients with uncomplicated duodenal ulceration, *H. pylori* eradication is clinically superior to traditional therapies and is cheaper. Evidence is beginning to emerge that these savings also occur in practice, although a minority (16–30%) of patients on long-term maintenance therapy for duodenal ulceration are unable to discontinue their acid-suppressing drugs after *H. pylori* eradication.

Chapter 7

Non-steroidal anti-inflammatory drugs and the gut

Introduction

Non-steroidal anti-inflammatory drugs (NSAIDs) are widely prescribed for musculoskeletal and joint problems, and they are associated with significant side-effects, many of which affect the gastrointestinal tract. Dyspepsia, epigastric pain, nausea and vomiting are the commonest symptoms associated with NSAID ingestion, which can also lead to gastric erosions, gastric and duodenal ulceration and ulcer haemorrhage and perforation. NSAIDs less commonly affect the small bowel, leading to changes similar to those found in inflammatory bowel disease. Co-prescription with an NSAID of a gastro-protective drug such as a proton pump inhibitor or prostaglandin agonist provides good protection against the gastroduodenal complications of NSAID therapy, even in patients with a history of previous peptic ulceration or NSAID-induced gastrointestinal haemorrhage.

Significance

NSAIDs account for around 5% of all prescribed medicines in this country. Their action depends on inhibition of cyclo-oxygenase pathways. Most currently used NSAIDs inhibit COX-1 pathways, but the more recently introduced COX-2 specific NSAIDs are associated with reduced gastrointestinal toxicity, although they are likely to be more expensive than many of the COX-1 drugs. Because dyspeptic symptoms are themselves so common, the prevalence of NSAID-induced symptoms is difficult to estimate, although there is general agreement that dyspepsia is more common in patients taking NSAIDs. However, the more serious complications of NSAID-induced gastrointestinal damage may not be preceded by symptoms, so both ulcer haemorrhage and perforation can occur in patients who have taken NSAIDs for some time without apparent problems.

Key clinical points

- In general terms, NSAIDs are more likely to cause problems in older patients and in those with concurrent serious disorders. Their prescription should therefore be considered carefully in these groups of patients.

- All patients who are prescribed NSAIDs should be advised to take them in accordance with the manufacturer's instructions for the particular drug, especially with regard to the relationship between dosing and mealtimes, and the need to report adverse effects and stop medication if these become persistent.

- Gastrointestinal toxicity is more likely to occur with combinations of more than one NSAID, with high dosages, and in combination with corticosteroids.

Key therapeutic points

- When NSAIDs are prescribed to older, higher-risk patients, a history of peptic ulceration or significant dyspeptic symptoms should suggest the co-prescription of a gastroprotective agent. Standard-dose proton pump inhibitor therapy is appropriate and effective, and is associated with fewer side-effects than are prostaglandin agonists such as misoprostol.

- Patients with an NSAID-related complication (i.e. perforation or haemorrhage) who require continued NSAID treatment should always receive co-prescription of a gastroprotective agent, as described above.

- In younger patients without digestive symptoms or a positive history of digestive disease, co-prescription is not generally recommended unless there is concomitant serious disease or the patient is taking other drugs which may contribute to gastrointestinal problems (e.g. steroids).

Guidelines

Dickson J *et al.* (1994) *Partnership in Practice – the Management of Osteoarthritis.* The Primary Care Rheumatology Society, Northallerton.

A Canadian evidence-based consensus guideline on the use of NSAIDs in musculoskeletal disease can be found at www.cma.ca/cmaj/vol-155/0077.htm

Access to services

Co-ordinated guidance from local gastroenterologists and rheumatologists on current prescribing policy may be helpful. Direct access to endoscopy may occasionally be required. Patients with gastrointestinal complications of NSAID therapy (peptic ulcer bleeding and perforation) are best cared for in a designated multidisciplinary unit.

Risk management

The prevalence and pattern of NSAID prescribing is a germane topic for practice audit. Specific aspects should include indications and contraindications, adverse events and the appropriateness of long-term therapy. A practice policy for cost-effective NSAID treatment and a practice formulary for NSAID drug selection and gastroprotective drug prescription should be generated.

Health economics

In the USA, one-third of the drug costs of arthritis treatment relate to gastrointestinal side-effects. The cost-effectiveness of widespread co-prescription of proton pump inhibitors and prostaglandin agonists (relatively expensive drugs) with NSAIDs in general practice remains controversial. Current recommendations are to restrict co-prescription to patients who are at demonstrably higher risk of complications. The availability of COX-2 NSAIDs will change the health economic picture by reducing the need for co-prescription of gastroprotective drugs.

Chapter 8

Haematemesis and melaena

Introduction

Haematemesis and melaena are events that signify bleeding from the upper gastrointestinal tract. They require prompt investigation and therapy.

Significance

The annual incidence of acute upper gastrointestinal haemorrhage is 103 in 100 000 adults, rising from 23 in 100 000 in those under 30 years of age to 485 in 100 000 in those over 75 years. Peptic ulcer disease is responsible for half of all cases. The mortality rate is 11%, with most deaths occurring in the elderly or those with co-morbidity. Most of these deaths occur among the 20% of patients who have severe bleeding from erosion of a major artery, and who require resuscitation and therapeutic intervention.

Key clinical points

- Patients with haematemesis and/or melaena require urgent admission to hospital for evaluation.

- NSAIDs are an important cause of haematemesis and melaena.

- There is evidence that specialised 'bleeding units' reduce mortality and make better use of resources than management by generalists working in conventional medical or surgical units.

- Endoscopy is the principal investigation. Its timing is dictated by the severity of bleeding and the patient's general condition.

Key therapeutic points

- Endoscopic therapies may use thermal or injection techniques. Effective thermal techniques use either a heater probe or multipolar electrocoagulation. Effective injection techniques use fibrin glue or thrombin. It is likely that a combination of thermal and injection techniques represents the best option.

- Following endoscopic treatment of bleeding peptic ulcer, a high-dose infusion of omeprazole substantially reduces the rate of re-bleeding.

- Patients who fail to respond to these measures require surgery to arrest the haemorrhage.

- Definitive surgical procedures for patients with treatable causes of peptic ulcer disease (*H. pylori* infection, NSAID use) should not be necessary.

Guidelines

Palmer KR and Choudari CP (1995) Endoscopic intervention in bleeding peptic ulcer. *Gut.* 37: 161–4.

Access to services

Units that accept emergency medical admissions should have a designated team consisting of gastroenterologists, surgeons and nurses who are experienced in the management of acute upper gastrointestinal haemorrhage.

Risk management

The use of NSAID drugs in patients with a history of dyspepsia and in the elderly requires careful consideration. Audit and review of the risks and benefits of NSAIDs in patients with these risk factors will contribute to risk minimisation.

Health economics

The incidence of acute gastrointestinal bleeding will rise with increasing longevity of the population. The potential to limit mortality, which relates mainly to age and comorbidity, is small.

Chapter 9

Upper gastrointestinal cancer

Definition

Cancers of the oesophagus, stomach and pancreas are referred to collectively as upper gastrointestinal cancers.

Significance

Upper gastrointestinal cancers account for 18 250 deaths annually in England and Wales (33 per year in a PCG of 100 000), and represent 13.5% of all cancer deaths. Survival is closely related to the stage of the disease at the time of diagnosis. Early cancers of the oesophagus and stomach (lesions confined to mucosa or sub-mucosa) have a 5-year survival in excess of 90%. With more advanced disease, the 5-year survival decreases to 30%. Many patients present with advanced disease. The incidence and mortality of gastric cancer are declining, but the incidence of adenocarcinoma of the oesophageal cardia is increasing significantly, and it is estimated that the number of cases will double in the next 10 years. The incidence rate of pancreatic cancer is stable.

Key clinical points

- The most important risk factors for upper gastrointestinal cancer are age and gender. Around 90% of cancers of the stomach and pancreas occur over the age of 55 years, and 90% of oesophageal cancers occur over the age of 40 years. All of them are more common in males.

- All patients with the alarm symptoms of weight loss, gastro-intestinal bleeding, anaemia, anorexia, abdominal mass or dysphagia, regardless of age, should be urgently investigated.

- All patients with new-onset symptoms of dyspepsia above the age of 45 years should be investigated by gastroscopy.

- Smoking, excessive alcohol consumption and poor diet are associated with an increased risk of upper gastrointestinal cancers. A positive family history, Barrett's oesophagus, pernicious anaemia, infection with *Helicobacter pylori* or previous gastric surgery also increase the risk.

- Patients with Barrett's oesophagus are offered 1- to 3-yearly surveillance endoscopy by most gastroenterologists. The evidence for this practice is conflicting, and a definitive study is still awaited.

- A GP with an average list will see less than one new upper gastrointestinal cancer each year.

Guidelines

British Society of Gastroenterology (1996) *Dyspepsia Management Guidelines*. British Society of Gastroenterology, London.

Many areas have local guidelines on referral to open-access endoscopy services.

Patient information can be found at
www.rex.nci.nih.gov/wtnk_pubs/stomach/index.htm

Access to services

Ready access to endoscopy is essential for the management of patients with upper gastrointestinal symptoms. Abdominal ultrasound facilities should also be available.

For patients with resectable disease there is wide variation in outcome following surgery. Referral should be to a unit that specialises in the treatment of upper gastrointestinal cancers, in accordance with Department of Health guidelines.

Risk management

Critical incident review can be undertaken after each new diagnosis.

Practices can audit their management and use of investigations in patients who present with upper abdominal symptoms. Data-recording of risk factors such as smoking, alcohol consumption and family history are also suitable topics for audit.

Health economics

Although there are direct costs associated with the treatment of upper gastrointestinal cancers, the principal arguments centre on the cost of investigations needed to increase the proportion of patients with early-stage disease at diagnosis.

Chapter 10

Gallstones

Introduction

Gallstones are accretions of cholesterol or pigment that develop within the gall-bladder. They affect up to 20% of the population, although 80% of cases are symptomless. They are twice as common in women as in men, particularly in the middle-aged, the multiparous and the obese.

Significance

Gallstones are most commonly manifested by biliary colic – a spasmodic pain caused by impaction of a stone in the gall-bladder neck, common bile duct or ampulla of Vater. The most frequent complication of gallstones is acute cholecystitis (inflammation secondary to obstruction of the cystic duct). Among asymptomatic individuals with gallstones there is a 1–2% annual rate of developing symptoms. There is a higher incidence of gallstones in diabetics, although this appears to be due to factors other than the diabetes. Diabetics become symptomatic at the same rate as members of the non-diabetic population.

Key clinical points

- Gallstones are common. In patients with upper abdominal symptoms who are found to have gallstones, a careful clinical history can help to distinguish between those for whom they are the cause and those in whom they are an incidental finding.

- Around 90% of patients with gallstones present with pain as the first manifestation. Only 10% first present with a biliary complication such as acute cholecystitis or pancreatitis.

- Diabetics who undergo emergency surgery for biliary complications experience increased morbidity (39% compared to 21% in non-diabetics).

- Once patients are symptomatic, there is a 6% annual rate of worsening symptoms or biliary complications.

Key therapeutic points

- Patients with symptomatic gallstones should be offered cholecystectomy.

- Patients with complications of gallstones (acute cholecystitis, choledocholithiasis, cholangitis, pancreatitis) should have early surgical treatment to prevent further complications.

- For elective procedures, laparoscopic cholecystectomy is as safe as open cholecystectomy. At 3 months, quality of life and satisfaction with scarring are equal. There is conflicting evidence that length of stay or recovery time may be shorter with the laparoscopic approach.

- Acute cholecystitis should be treated with early cholecystectomy. In this situation, the laparoscopic approach is at least as safe as the open approach, and has the benefit of a shorter hospital stay.

- Endoscopic retrograde cholangiopancreatography (ERCP) and sphincterotomy/stone extraction are valuable in the management of gallstone pancreatitis and choledocholithiasis.

- Dissolution therapy is now rarely used. It takes 1–2 years and is only suitable for the minority of patients who have small radiolucent stones within a functioning gall-bladder. The stone recurrence rate at 5 years is 30–50%.

- Extracorporeal shock-wave lithotripsy is suitable for patients with a single large radiolucent stone. It is associated with severe side-effects (pancreatitis, cholecystitis) in 3–5% of cases and has a 9% risk of recurrence at 1 year.

Guidelines

Information for doctors is available at www.netdoctor.co.uk
    Patient information from the Leeds Institute for Minimally Invasive Therapy is available at www.limit.ac.uk/gallstones.htm

Access to services

Ultrasound examination of the biliary tract is the investigation of choice for gallstones, and it should be freely available to GPs.
    Surgical services with training and experience in laparoscopic as

well as open biliary tract surgery should be locally available. Gastroenterology services with ERCP expertise should also be locally available.

Risk management

Audit of the management of patients who develop complications of gallstones.

Health economics

A PCG population will have about 75 cholecystectomies each year. After considering both perioperative and hospitalisation costs, a cost-minimisation analysis found that laparoscopic cholecystectomy was significantly more expensive than the open procedure (£1486 compared to £1090). However, other studies have found that indirect cost savings, earlier discharge and earlier return to work swing the balance in favour of laparoscopic surgery. The widespread perception that laparoscopic surgery is the more acceptable alternative is an obstacle to its rigorous validation.

Chapter 11

Viral hepatitis

Definition

Viral hepatitis is inflammation of the liver resulting from infection, usually by one of the hepatitis viruses, the commonest of which are the hepatitis A, B and C viruses. Their clinical manifestations are similar in the acute phase, but there are important differences in their modes of transmission and in long-term prognosis.

Significance

Hepatitis A virus (HAV) is spread by faecal–oral contamination. Hepatitis B virus (HBV) is spread sexually and by contact with infected blood and body fluids. Hepatitis C virus (HCV) is spread principally by blood and infected needles. Although a significant minority of cases of hepatitis C have become infected through the transfusion of blood or blood products prior to the introduction of screening processes, most cases result from intravenous drug abuse. Up to 70% of intravenous drug users are seropositive for HCV.

HAV causes a self-limiting illness and rarely has long-term sequelae. It is a risk for travellers to developing countries. Acute infection with HBV is a debilitating condition which may require hospitalisation, whereas HCV infection can go unnoticed. Chronic hepatitis follows in 5–10% of cases of HBV and in 85% of cases of HCV, and carries the risk of cirrhosis and hepatocellular carcinoma. The prevalence of HBV and HCV infection varies considerably between ethnic and other social groups. Accurate data for HCV prevalence are not available, but it is estimated that there may be up to 100 carrriers per 100 000 members of the population in the UK.

Key clinical points

- Vaccination against HAV is safe and effective.

- For HBV there is a risk of mother-to-child spread during the neonatal period, which then carries an 80% risk of chronic hepatitis.

- The rate of progression of chronic HBV infection to cirrhosis is 10–40% over 10 or more years, and the rate of neoplastic transformation of HBV cirrhosis is 3–6% per year.

- HBV vaccination is safe and effective. The lifetime risk of HBV infection can be reduced by 70% by neonatal vaccination, or by 45% by adolescent vaccination.

- Chronic HCV infection results in abnormal alanine aminotransferase (ALT) levels in 75% of cases. Of these, two-thirds will run a relatively benign, slowly progressive course. The remaining third, who are most accurately identified as having moderate or severe hepatitis by the presence of marked necro-inflammatory changes and fibrosis on liver biopsy, carry a high risk of developing cirrhosis over a period of 10 years.

- The risk of developing hepatocellular carcinoma in the HCV cirrhotic patient is 1–5% per year.

- End-stage cirrhosis due to HCV is the most common indication for liver transplantation.

Key therapeutic points

- Factors that accelerate liver disease, such as alcohol abuse, should be discussed with the patient who has chronic hepatitis.

- Interferon therapy for chronic HBV infection results in long-term 'cure', as demonstrated by surrogate markers, in 25% of patients. The duration of therapy required is dependent on the HBV variant.

- There is no acceptable evidence for a protective effect of interferon against development of hepatocellular carcinoma in HBV-related cirrhosis.

- Treatment of HCV with interferon can stop viral replication and reduce associated morbidity and mortality. It is indicated for acute HCV infection and for treatment of patients with moderate to severe chronic hepatitis. Its benefits in patients with histologically mild disease are uncertain.

- Combination therapy with interferon and ribavirin increases the percentage of HCV patients who show a sustained response to treatment to about 40%, but fails to reduce the number of non-responders significantly.

Guidelines

A customised Medline service is available at
http://medlineplus.nlm.nih.gov/medlineplus/hepatitis.html
   Patient information is available at
www.hebs.scot.nhs.uk/hiv/hivphep.htm
   Information on travel vaccination is available at
www.axl.co.uk/scieh/

Access to services

Laboratory services for the serological diagnosis of the full range of acute and chronic hepatitis virus infections should be readily available.

The services of a gastroenterologist with expertise in the management of liver disease should also be readily available.

Risk management

- In line with Department of Health recommendations, practices should have an agreed policy on the identification of at-risk groups and the offering of HAV and/or HBV vaccination to those groups.

- Practices should agree a policy on the identification and screening of at-risk patients for HCV infection.

Health economics

- The cost of treating one case of chronic HCV infection is £3000–6000 per annum. The treatment of 1000 patients will save about 25 lives.

- The incremental cost-effectiveness rate for use of interferon in HBV and HCV is in the region of £15 000 per year of life saved.

- The average cost of liver transplantation for HCV infection is £32 000–£45 000, to which must be added the costs of long-term antiviral therapy.

Chapter 12

Coeliac disease

Introduction

Coeliac disease is a chronic inflammatory disorder that affects the mucosa of the small intestine and is triggered by a sensitivity to gluten. This results in villous atrophy and malabsorption.

Significance

One in 300 members of the population is affected by coeliac disease, with as many as two-thirds of cases going undetected. A PCG would expect to have about 330 cases. In childhood, coeliac disease can result in failure to thrive and growth problems. However, it is now more commonly seen in adults, in whom the classical symptoms are often absent.

Because coeliac disease often causes non-specific symptoms, it may go undiagnosed for long periods of time. Nevertheless, it has significant associated long-term morbidity, which can be reversed with appropriate treatment. For this reason, a high index of suspicion of coeliac disease is justified in patients with unexplained or non-specific symptoms.

Key clinical points

- The diagnosis should be considered in cases of unexplained diarrhoea, iron or folate deficiency anaemia, chronic fatigue or infertility.

- There is an increased likelihood of the condition if there is a family history of coeliac disease, and in patients with insulin-dependent diabetes, autoimmune thyroid disease, osteoporosis or undefined neurological disorders.

- The endomysial antibody test is the initial investigation of choice, with a sensitivity of 86% and specificity of 100%. Patients who test positive should be offered endoscopy and intestinal biopsy.

- Long-term complications include osteoporosis and a twofold increase in the risk of gastrointestinal tumours (small-bowel adenocarcinoma and enteropathy-associated T-cell lymphoma).

- Bone mineral density should be measured at the time of diagnosis and then again at the menopause (in women), at age 55 years (in men), or in the event of a fragility fracture.

Key therapeutic points

- The primary treatment is with a strict and lifelong gluten-free diet, and GPs are often asked to prescribe these products.

- Long-term compliance protects against symptomatic disease, osteoporosis and gastrointestinal malignancy.

- Supplements of deficient nutrients, iron, folic acid and calcium may be required.

- Dietitians have a key role in the management of coeliac disease.

Guidelines

Primary Care Society for Gastroenterology (1999) *Decision Points in the Management of Adult Coeliac Disease in Primary Care.* Primary Care Society for Gastroenterology, Oxford; www.pcsg.org.uk

Patient information can be obtained from the Coeliac Society of the UK, PO Box 220, High Wycombe, Bucks HP11 2HY; www.coeliac.co.uk

Access to services

GPs should have access to endomysial antibody tests. Primary healthcare teams should be supported by a dietetic service with expertise in the dietary management of coeliac disease.

Risk management

Many patients with coeliac disease are lost to follow-up. Practices can set up recall systems for regular review. Performance indicators for the review include bone mineral density testing at agreed intervals, and the provision of dietetic advice. A case-finding approach can be used in populations at increased risk (e.g. in individuals with a family history, associated conditions, osteoporosis, infertility or chronic fatigue).

Health economics

The cost of prescribing gluten-free products in England in 1998 was £13.8 million. However, the true cost to the individual is likely to be higher, as some products may be bought 'over the counter'. The average annual cost of prescriptions for gluten-free foods is estimated to be £600 per patient.

The cost savings from preventing fragility fractures and gastro-intestinal malignancies have not been quantified, but they are likely to be significant.

Chapter 13

Irritable bowel syndrome

Introduction

Irritable bowel syndrome (IBS) is a condition in which recurrent abdominal pain is associated with a change in bowel habit and abdominal bloating. The precise pathological mechanisms involved in IBS are poorly understood, and there is no 'gold-standard' diagnostic test, so the diagnosis has to be made on the basis of the clinical history and the pattern and combination of symptoms. For many years the Manning criteria were used as a guide to diagnosis. More recently, specialist working groups have elaborated the Rome I and Rome II criteria for the diagnosis of IBS, although at present these are more useful for selecting patients in research studies than for making a diagnosis in general practice. IBS sufferers are generally divided into three main types, namely diarrhoea-predominant, constipation-predominant and alternating types. Pain and bloating are features of all three types.

Significance

Symptoms compatible with a clinical diagnosis of IBS are reported by 10–22% of subjects sampled from the general population in most European countries. Lower bowel symptoms account for 4–5% of consultations in primary care, and many of these patients will have IBS. Functional digestive disorders, including IBS, account for up to one-third of all referrals and half of all patients attending for follow-up appointments in gastroenterology clinics. Although IBS is not a life-threatening condition, it has a considerable negative impact on patients' quality of life, and can result in inappropriate and excessive investigation and referral for specialist opinions. There is a complex interaction between life events, psychological state and the symptoms of IBS.

Key clinical points

- IBS is defined by the Rome II criteria as the presence for at least 12 weeks (which need not be consecutive) in the preceding 12 months of abdominal discomfort or pain that has two of the following three features:
    relieved with defaecation
    onset associated with a change in frequency of stool
    onset associated with a change in form (appearance) of stool.

- Only about one-third of IBS patients consult general practitioners; anxiety and depression and concern about the seriousness of their symptoms are important reasons for consultation.

- A change in bowel habit can, of course, be an early warning of large bowel cancer. If this symptom is accompanied by any other alarm symptoms, such as weight loss, evidence of bleeding, anaemia or systemic illness, particularly in patients in middle age and beyond, prompt investigation should be undertaken.

- In younger patients, particularly when there is persistent bloody diarrhoea or pain, the possibility of inflammatory bowel disease should also be considered.

- A diagnosis based on symptoms, rather than on the exclusion of serious disease, should be the goal in low-risk patients who do not fall into the alarm categories mentioned above, although a careful physical examination is always important. If there is doubt, a full blood count and erythrocyte sedimentation rate (ESR) may be helpful, but no other routine investigations are recommended. A small proportion of patients with IBS may have lactose intolerance.

- A sympathetically taken history and a clear explanation and account of the likely course of the disease are likely to be more efficacious in management than investigation and referral, unless these are dictated by physician uncertainty or patient pressures.

- Although anxiety and depression are not part of IBS *per se*, a careful mental state examination should be conducted in patients with troublesome symptoms.

- IBS is a long-term problem, with frequent exacerbations and remissions. Patients may require repeated reassurance that their symptoms do not signify serious disease, but changing symptoms and the development of any of the alarm symptoms mentioned above should lead to a heightened level of diagnostic suspicion of more serious, organic disease.

Key therapeutic points

- Management depends on a shared understanding of the condition, appropriate dietary advice and trials of therapy.

- Fibre is not a panacea, and it can make diarrhoea-predominant IBS worse.

- Lactose malabsorption is present in up to 25% of patients with IBS, and those with a positive lactose intolerance test should eliminate lactose from their diet.

- Tricyclic antidepressants produce a significant improvement in symptoms through their neuromodulatory and analgesic properties.

- Loperamide is effective in reducing the number of stools in diarrhoea-predominant IBS.

- Anti-spasmodic drugs are of some value in certain patients, although they are often relatively ineffective. New agents such as $5HT_3$- and $5HT_4$-antagonists and agonists are currently under development and will soon be available. These may offer more reliable symptom relief.

- Psychological interventions are beneficial in patients who are likely to respond to these approaches, namely those under the age of 50 years who have insight about the role of stressors and who have lower anxiety levels. Hypnosis has been shown to be effective in randomised controlled trials, although it is relatively expensive in terms of time and expertise.

Guidelines

The American Gastroenterology Association medical position statement is a useful clinical guideline, although it is more interventionist than is usual in UK practice. Details are available at www.wbsaunders.com/gastro/policy/v112n6p2118.html

Patient information is available at www.ibscentral.com

Access to services

Most investigations and referrals associated with IBS – for problem patients or unusual symptoms – are generally routinely available at district hospitals. However, particularly difficult patients may require referral to specialist centres with a particular interest in IBS, in which a multidisciplinary approach involving psychologists and psychiatrists as well as gastroenterologists is employed.

Risk management

Note the review of patients with IBS in order to determine the use of investigations and out-patient referrals. Critical incident analysis of new diagnoses of colon cancer and inflammatory bowel disease is useful, since a number of these patients may initially be misdiagnosed as having irritable bowel syndrome.

Health economics

IBS costs the NHS approximately £45 million each year, with the costs being equally divided between consultations in general practice, hospital out-patient appointments and drug therapy. These costs are likely to be reduced if positive symptom-based diagnoses are made more frequently in primary care, and if reassurance and explanation can be backed up by the availability of reliably effective drug therapy.

Patients with IBS incur total annual healthcare costs that are 70% higher than those for patients without IBS.

Chapter 14

Inflammatory bowel disease

Introduction

Ulcerative colitis (UC) and Crohn's disease (CD) are the principal non-specific inflammatory bowel diseases. UC primarily affects the mucosa and submucosa of the colon, whereas CD may affect any part of the gastrointestinal tract and involves all layers of the intestinal wall. Both diseases are idiopathic and commonly run a chronic relapsing course.

Significance

The most recent data indicate an incidence of inflammatory bowel disease (IBD) of around 20 in 100 000 per year in the UK, the ratio of UC to CD being between 2:1 and 3:1. The incidence of both diseases is now stable and the associated mortality is low. As a result, around 1% of the population will suffer one or more prolonged episodes of IBD in their lifetime.

Key clinical points

- Inflammatory bowel disease should be considered in patients with diarrhoea (bloody or otherwise) that persists for more than 2 weeks in the absence of any identifiable pathogen.

- Adequate assessment requires endoscopy and mucosal biopsy, or sometimes radiological studies in the case of Crohn's disease. Disease activity can be quantified clinically and by laboratory tests.

- Patients in whom IBD is suspected should be referred for specialist assessment.

- Patients with ulcerative colitis extending beyond the left colon should be reviewed periodically in a specialist clinic. Those with disease of more than 10 years' duration should be offered colonoscopic surveillance for mucosal dysplasia or early colonic cancer.

- Symptom relapse in patients with left-sided or extensive colitis requires prompt action. Those who are well and pass less than 6 stools per day are likely to require steroids in doses of 20–40 mg daily, together with specialist review. For those who are ill, admission to hospital is more appropriate.

Key therapeutic points

- Corticosteroids are the principal drugs used to induce remission for both UC and CD, but they are not normally used for long-term maintenance therapy. Once remission has been induced, oral aminosalicylates substantially reduce the relapse rate for UC but are less effective in CD. Both diseases may respond to azathioprine.

- The newer aminosalicylates, e.g. mesalazine, are safer and more tolerable, and are to be preferred when initiating treatment.

- Cyclosporin is of limited effectiveness in UC, and is ineffective in CD.

- Oral budesonide is comparable to oral steroids in inducing remission in active ileocaecal Crohn's disease, but causes fewer corticosteroid side-effects. Its safety and effectiveness as a long-term therapy have not been determined.

- Tumour necrosis factor (TNF-alpha) plays an important pathogenic role in Crohn's disease. A single infusion of infliximab, a monoclonal antibody to TNF-alpha, will induce remission in 33% of patients with refractory active disease. Successful healing of more than 50% of perianal fistulae has been reported in 62% of patients treated with three infusions of infliximab.

Guidelines

British Society of Gastroenterology (1996) *Inflammatory Bowel Disease. BSG Guidelines in Gastroenterology.* British Society of Gastroenterology, London.

Patient group details and further information are available from the National Association for Colitis and Crohn's Disease at www.nacc.org.uk

Access to services

- Patients with IBD are ideally managed by a specialist gastro-enterology team with a specific interest in inflammatory bowel disease. The long-term care of these patients is eminently suited to a shared-care approach with the primary healthcare team.

- Specialist clinics should provide rapid access for patients with symptom relapse. Quality initiatives in this area include direct phone lines and open access to clinics.

Risk management

- Systems should be in place to ensure that patients on long-term aminosalicylate therapy undergo annual monitoring of liver and renal function.

- A management protocol for IBD relapse should be jointly agreed between the GP and the specialist, and shared with the patient. This should define relapse, the immediate therapy to be given and the specialist response.

- All patients with a history of extensive UC for 10 years or more should be offered colonoscopic surveillance.

Health economics

Up to 30% of patients with left-sided or extensive colitis are not under specialist care.

Two USA studies have demonstrated that lower-cost medications have a relatively small effect on the overall cost of illness. Drug therapies that are capable of reducing rates of hospitalisation or surgery could lower the total costs considerably. IBD has significant long-term personal costs in terms of quality of life and number of working days lost.

A single infusion of infliximab costs approximately £450.

Chapter 15

Gastroenteritis

Introduction

Gastroenteritis is inflammation of the gastrointestinal tract characterised by nausea, vomiting and diarrhoea, often with abdominal pain and pyrexia. It may lead to dehydration and hypotension.

Significance

Gastroenteritis causes significant morbidity among children and the elderly. Although only 1 in 6 adults consult their doctor about the condition, in children 15 in 1000 cases are admitted to hospital each year. A population of 100 000 would have generated 202 public health notifications of food poisoning in 1998, a figure that has doubled in the past 10 years.

In an average PCG, 40 children might be admitted with

gastroenteritis each year. The number of deaths from diarrhoeal disease in children has decreased from 340 to 20 per year over the past 20 years (in England and Wales), mainly due to management with oral rehydration therapy (ORT).

Key clinical points

- Gastroenteritis is usually caused by an ingested infectious agent, and less often by bacterial or chemical toxins.

- In a UK research study of gastroenteritis in the community, no causative organism was isolated in over 50% of cases.

- Most cases are contracted from food or water, and should be classified as food poisoning. There is a statutory requirement to notify cases to the local Director of Public Health.

- Breastfeeding in the first 4–6 months of life protects against non-viral pathogens.

- Admission to hospital should be considered for children who have bloody diarrhoea or who are 7% or more dehydrated (indicated by obvious loss of skin tone, sunken eyes, marked thirst/oliguria, restlessness or apathy).

Key therapeutic points

- Both adults and children should use ORT to correct fluid and electrolyte losses in the acute phase. In one study of children admitted to hospital, less than two-thirds had been given ORT in primary care.

- Cereal-based ORT (Dioralyte Relief) significantly reduces stool volume, as does early refeeding.

- Unrestricted diets do not worsen the course or symptoms of mild diarrhoea, and can decrease stool output. Children with diarrhoea who are not dehydrated should be fed an age-appropriate diet. Those who are dehydrated should be fed as soon as they have been rehydrated.

- Parental understanding of the disease and instructions for therapy are crucially important.

- Drug therapies (e.g. anticholinergics, adsorbents, loperamide) are not recommended in the treatment of acute diarrhoea in children.

- Post-infective diarrhoea is common, and these days is not normally due to lactose intolerance.

- Antibiotic therapy is appropriate if there is a strong suspicion of or proven bacterial infection – for example, *Salmonella* bacteraemia (ciprofloxacin), *Campylobacter* (erythromycin or ciprofloxacin), *Shigella* (ciprofloxacin), traveller's diarrhoea (trimethoprim, doxycycline or ciprofloxacin).

- Parents should be discouraged from using non-physiological rehydration solutions such as Lucozade or Coca-Cola.

Guidelines

Anon (1996) Practice parameter: the management of acute gastroenteritis in young children. *Paediatrics.* **97**: 424–35.

Guidelines for the control of infectious diseases (*The Blue Book*) are available at
http://hna.ffh.vic.gov.au/phb/hprot/inf_dis/bluebook/index.htm
Patient information is available at
www.ridgeway-surgery.demon.co.uk/newslett/gastroen.htm

Access to services

Laboratory services for the isolation of causative pathogens should be readily available to GPs.

Risk management – possible audit topics for PCGs/PCTs

In adults, possible topics include the following:

- mapping of recorded cases at practice level with notifications to the local Director of Public Health

- use of antibiotics for diarrhoeal illness.

In children, possible topics include the following:

- all members of the primary healthcare team should be aware of modern oral rehydration therapy and refeeding practices

- practice protocol for gastroenteritis in children

- case review of all admissions to hospital with nausea/vomiting as critical incident analysis to identify learning points for dissemination to the primary healthcare team.

Health economics

The cost of prescribing ORT in England in 1998 was £2.7 million. The hospital costs of in-patient treatment for infectious intestinal disease average £769 per episode.

Chapter 16

Constipation

Introduction

Constipation is a condition in which bowel evacuations occur infrequently, or in which the faeces are small and hard, or where passage of faeces causes difficulty or pain. The frequency of bowel evacuation varies considerably from one person to another, and the normal state cannot be precisely defined.

Significance

Among adults in the UK, 10% strain at stool at least 25% of the time, and 1% pass fewer than 2 stools per week. Constipation is more prevalent among women and in the elderly, of whom up to 25% have self-reported constipation. Using the Rome criteria for diagnosis of constipation, the prevalence in women aged 25–69 years is 8.2%.

Key clinical points

- Functional constipation is by far the commonest cause, due to inadequate fibre intake, pregnancy, old age or idiopathic slow transit.

- Other causes include drug side-effects and rare causes such as structural abnormalities, neurological, endocrine or metabolic disorders, and depression.

- Digital examination of the rectum is an important part of the assessment, and will often reveal a large faecal mass in the rectum.

- Measurement of whole-gut transit time is useful in adults, although half of those referred to hospital because of constipation have a normal transit time.

Key therapeutic points

- The initial goal of treatment in adults is to empty the rectum. The aim is to then develop a regular bowel habit using diet together with regular and continuous laxatives to keep the stool soft.

- Observational studies suggest that dietary fibre is effective in preventing constipation, although this has not been confirmed by randomised controlled trials. Although some patients find that increasing dietary fibre increases abdominal pain and distension, most cases are helped by a diet containing 20–30 g of fibre per day, derived from wholemeal bread, breakfast cereals, fruit and vegetables.

- Most of the placebo-controlled trials of laxatives in adults have been small and show a non-significant trend in favour of treatment. There have been few direct comparisons between different classes of laxatives, and there is little evidence of any benefit of combinations of drugs.

- In the absence of evidence to the contrary, it appears sensible to start drug therapy using the cheapest preparation. Drugs should be continued for a period of 4 weeks in order to assess their potential for benefit.

- There is no evidence that danthron laxatives are more effective than other preparations, and they should not be routinely used in the treatment of constipation.

- Slow-transit constipation is seen mainly in women, with intervals of a week or more between bowel movements. The condition is resistant to dietary measures, and most patients make intermittent use of stimulant laxatives. If it is intractable, total colectomy with ileorectal anastamosis will restore normal bowel function to 50% of these patients, but a minority – often those with psychiatric disturbances – will continue to complain of constipation.

Guidelines

Petticrew M *et al.* (1997) Systematic review of the effectiveness of laxatives in the elderly. *Health Technology Assessment.* 1(13): 1–52. www.hta.nhsweb.nhs.uk/fullmono/mon113.pdf

Access to services

- Dietetic advice is an important resource in the management of constipation, and should be available in primary care.

- A specialist centre with a specific interest in constipation should be identified for the management of intractable constipation.

Risk management

- Systems should be in place to monitor the long-term prescription of laxative drugs and to ensure that they continue to be appropriate.

Health economics

- Although it is often considered to be a trivial problem, constipation is responsible for 450 000 general practitioner consultations per year in England and Wales.

- Treatments for constipation account for prescription costs of £47 million annually in England alone.

Chapter 17

Minor anal conditions

Introduction

Minor anal conditions include haemorrhoids, anal fissure, fistula in ano, pruritus ani and perianal warts. Haemorrhoids are caused principally by constipation and straining, although their onset in women may be associated with pregnancy. Fissure is most commonly seen in younger patients. It is often associated with anal sphincter spasm, but may also arise as a result of local trauma, as might occur in anal intercourse. The more common causes of pruritus ani include poor hygiene, anal pathology (haemorrhoids, fissure, fistula), infections, skin disorders and drug sensitivities. Condylomata acuminata are caused by infection with human papillomavirus.

Significance

Minor anal conditions are common in the community. It is likely that they are the cause of a significant proportion of the rectal bleeding reported in community prevalence studies, where annual rates of the order of 15% are described. The annual consultation rate for piles and anal disorders in general practice is 1500 in 100 000.

Key clinical and therapeutic points

Haemorrhoids

- The cardinal symptom of haemorrhoids is fresh rectal bleeding which may be copious and may occur at the end of defaecation. Prolapse and discomfort caused by engorgement can also occur.

- Most haemorrhoids respond to an increase in dietary fibre and prevention of constipation and straining.

- There is no good quality evidence for the benefit of soothing local preparations, whether or not they contain a steroid, in treating haemorrhoids.

- Rubber-band ligation is the recommended initial treatment for all grades of haemorrhoids except those which are permanently prolapsed.

- Although haemorrhoidectomy shows a better response, it is associated with more complications and pain, and should therefore be reserved for those cases which fail to respond to rubber-band ligation. Manual dilatation of the anus, sclerotherapy and infra-red coagulation are all less effective.

Anal fissure

- Anal fissure is the commonest cause of pain (often searing in nature) on defaecation. This can be accompanied by slight fresh rectal bleeding, which is commonly noted on the toilet-paper.

- Anal fissure will often respond to stool softeners and analgesics. Nitroglycerin ointment 0.2% is effective in decreasing anal sphincter tone, and results in healing in 50% of cases. However, it is not presently available as a commercial preparation in community pharmacies.

- Chronic fissure that does not respond to these measures is treated surgically by lateral anal sphincterotomy.

Anal fistula

- Anal fistulas commonly present with recurrent perianal discharge, and are classified according to their position relative to the anal sphincter.

- Treatment of anal fistula is surgical, and at its simplest consists of laying open and curetting the track, and leaving it to heal by secondary intention.

- Antibiotics are ineffective in the treatment of anal fistula.

Pruritus ani

- Treatment measures for pruritus ani include careful washing of the area with water only, gentle but thorough drying, avoidance of scratching, avoiding the use of topical preparations and treatment of the underlying cause.

Perianal warts

- Treatment options for perianal warts include chemical methods (podophyllin), electrocautery or diathermy. Simple scissor excision is effective in 75% of cases.

Guidelines

None are available.

Access to services

Nitroglycerin ointment (0.2%) should be available as a commercial preparation on FP10 prescription.

Open-access flexible sigmoidoscopy services and rapid-access rectal bleeding clinics facilitate the prompt and accurate evaluation of rectal bleeding.

Risk management

Adequate assessment of patients in order to make a positive diagnosis of a minor anal condition is important. Factors that contribute to inadequate assessment include lack of a chaperone and lack of suitable examination facilities (i.e. separate examination room, surgical gloves, proctoscope).

Health economics

An average PCG can expect 75 patients to require specialist treatment for haemorrhoids over a 12-month period.

The annual cost of local haemorrhoid preparations to an average PCG in England is £14 500.

Chapter 18

Colorectal cancer

Introduction

Colorectal or large bowel cancer (CRC) is a malignant disorder that arises from the mucosa of the colon or rectum. Most CRCs evolve from adenomatous polyps. The time taken for transformation from polyp to invasive cancer is estimated to be 10 years.

Significance

CRC causes 19 000 deaths per annum in the UK, and is the second most common cause of cancer death. There are about 30 000 new cases each year, so that each GP is likely to see one new case per year. An average PCG will have 50 new cases per year.

Around 70% of CRCs arise in the rectum, sigmoid and descending colon, 75% present in patients over the age of 60 years, and 25% of cases present as emergencies. The overall 5-year survival rates in the UK have not improved significantly in recent decades and at 40% are among the worst in Europe, significantly lower than those in the USA.

The lifetime risk of developing CRC is 1 in 50, but the risk is significantly increased if:

- two or more first-degree relatives have CRC

- one first-degree relative aged < 45 years has CRC

- a patient has colonic adenomatous polyps > 1 cm in diameter

- a patient has longstanding extensive inflammatory bowel disease.

In over 75% of cases, inherited factors appear to be relatively unimportant, and most of these cases will be elderly (over 70 years of age). The most important environmental factor is diet.

Key clinical points

- Alarm symptoms include rectal bleeding, any unexplained alteration in bowel habit, tenesmus, abdominal pain, unexplained anaemia, faecal incontinence, anorexia and weight loss.

- Patients with persistent symptoms at any age require investigation by colonoscopy or flexible sigmoidoscopy and barium enema.

- The risk of CRC increases with age, but the disease is rare in individuals under the age of 45 years.

- In patients over 50 years of age, recent-onset rectal bleeding should not be attributed to haemorrhoids without first excluding CRC or an adenomatous polyp.

- Genetic advice should be sought for patients with a high-risk family history.

Management

- Multidisciplinary teams should manage the patient with CRC. These teams should have adopted high-quality clinical guidelines, and they should include a specialist colorectal cancer nurse.

- Pre-operative radiotherapy for rectal (but not colonic) cancer results in a 40% reduction in local recurrence.

- Adjuvant chemotherapy can increase the survival rate by at least 5% in Dukes B and C CRC.

- There is insufficient evidence available with regard to the value of long-term routine follow-up in detecting possible recurrence or progression. Most patients with symptoms consult their GP first. GP and hospital clinic follow-up have been found to be equally satisfactory.

Guidelines

Primary Care Society for Gastroenterology (1998) *Guidelines on the Early Detection of CRC in Primary Care.* Primary Care Society for Gastroenterology, Oxford; www.pcsg.org.uk/pcsgcolorect.htm

NHS Executive (1997) *Improving Outcomes in Colorectal Cancer.* NHS Executive, London; www.doh.gov.uk/canc/colrec.htm or NHS response line 0541 555455.

Patient information is available from the Cancer Research Campaign at www.crc.org.uk/cancer/aboutcan_common3.html

Access to services

GPs should have easy access to lower gastrointestinal endoscopy.

The estimated service requirement for colonoscopy is 0.5% of the population per annum. At present, 0.1% undergo colonoscopy annually.

Access to genetic assessment services is necessary for the evaluation of patients with a high-risk family history.

Risk management – possible audit topics for PCGs

- Quality indicators for endoscopic and surgical services should be monitored. These include waiting-times, completion rates for colonoscopy, surgical results and recurrence rates.

- Critical incident analysis of the interval between onset of symptoms and diagnosis (practice/PCG level).

- Quality of family history-taking at practice level, together with actions taken in response to positive findings.

- Patients with an adenomatous polyp more than 1 cm in diameter should have colonoscopic surveillance at 5-yearly intervals.

- Patients with a high-risk family history of CRC should have 3-yearly screening colonoscopy starting at age 40 years, or 10 years before the index case.

Health economics

- A PCG will spend about £500 000 a year on in-patient treatment for CRC.

- One case of CRC costs £4500 to investigate and treat.

- Faecal occult blood screening might cost £115 000 per life saved (incurring costs of £40 million per 3800 lives saved per year).

- Flexible sigmoidoscopy screening might cost £8500 per cancer death prevented.

- Cervical-screening or breast-screening programmes cost £30 000–50 000 per cancer death prevented.

Chapter 19

Stomas

Introduction

A gastrointestinal stoma is an artificial opening of the bowel on to the external skin. The commonest types of stoma are colostomy and ileostomy.

Significance

There are currently over 80 000 individuals in the UK with a stoma, and 22 000 new stomas are created each year. A PCG will have about 135 stoma patients and 37 new patients a year. Permanent stomas account for 65% of these, although surgical advances have increased the proportion of temporary stomas.

Key clinical points

- Stoma formation rates for rectal cancer are in the range 8–43% for different centres.

- If a patient is likely to be given a stoma (whether temporary or permanent), its nature and implications should be carefully explained to the patient and their carers, and its position should be discussed before surgery.

- Stomas are associated with disordered body image and impaired social and sexual functioning.

- Emotional problems, including depression, may affect up to 50% of patients with stomas.

Management

- Stoma patients are best managed by a specialised stoma-care nurse functioning as part of a multidisciplinary team.

- Most stoma patients use a stoma-care appliance (bag). These are one- or two-piece and may be disposable. The choice of appliance is best made by the patient in consultation with a stoma nurse. Patients with a sigmoid end colostomy may be suitable for management using irrigation.

- Dietary modification among ostomates is common. Clinicians should be aware of the effects of certain foods and drugs on stoma function, and of the need to avoid nutritional deficiencies.

- Employment capacity may be affected, and patients may need support from their GPs in their dealings with employers with regard to sanitary arrangements.

Guidelines

Details of the British Colostomy Association (BCA) are available at
www.bcass.org.uk
   Details of the International Ostomy Association, which provides
guidance and advice for all ostomates, are available at
www.ostomyinternational.org/
   Details of the Ileostomy and Internal Pouch Support Group (IA)
are available at www.ileostomypouch.demon.co.uk/

Access to services

- Specialist stoma-care nurses should be available to all ostomates
  locally. It is reported that 43% of specialist nurses are spon-
  sored by appliance manufacturers. This is likely to influence the
  product brands prescribed.

- Standardised information should be available to patients,
  including audio-tapes and videos, as well as written information, especially for the elderly.

Risk management

- Annual review of ostomates should be conducted in conjunction with the local stoma-care nurse.

- A review of the prescription of appliances, their types and
  quantities, and the use of ancillary items should be a part of this
  process.

- Patient satisfaction questionnaires and quality-of-life measures
  should be used.

Health economics

In 1998, the UK net ingredient cost of dispensing stoma appliances in the community was £92 million. This is equivalent to £150 000 per PCG per annum.

Chapter 20

Horizon scanning

Epidemiology

The epidemiology of peptic ulcer disease changed constantly during the twentieth century, and there is no reason to believe that this trend will not continue. *Helicobacter pylori* is increasingly being identified and eradicated, while improvements in social conditions have resulted in a progressive decline in its community acquisition and prevalence. As a result, duodenal ulcer is becoming a relatively uncommon condition, while the prevalence of gastro-oesophageal reflux symptoms and the diagnosis of gastro-oesophageal reflux disease are both rising rapidly. Rates of gastro-oesophageal cancer are rising faster than any other cancer rates, and gastric cancer itself seems to be declining in frequency. The incidence of colorectal cancer in Western societies appears to be relatively stable at present. It is likely that the incidence and complication rates of hepatitis B and C will continue to rise, and they pose increasing problems for management and the use of healthcare resources. In some communities, hepatitis C virus infection is present in up to 70% of intravenous drug users. This should be contrasted to an HIV prevalence of only 2% in the same communities.

Screening

The future of screening for colorectal cancer is uncertain. The randomised controlled trials of faecal occult blood testing have shown that mortality from CRC can be reduced by 15%, and pilot sites have now been established in the UK to test this screening modality further. However, a large and expensive trial of one-off flexible sigmoidoscopy is now in progress, but will not report for another 3–4 years. Of enormous potential interest are non-invasive imaging techniques which could possibly take the place of both occult blood testing and endoscopic screening. Virtual colonoscopy, using spiral CT and spiral MRI, is becoming a reality, and it is possible that a high-resolution image of the colon may be obtained non-invasively in a matter of minutes using these emerging technologies.

New technologies

In endoscopy, two developments are likely to change the way in which the procedure is regarded in the future. The first of these is the development of very small-bore, high-resolution endoscopes which can be inserted transnasally, permitting excellent and rapid assessment of the upper gastrointestinal tract with minimal distress to the patient and almost no need for sedation or anaesthesia. The second is the development of high-magnification endoscopy, which generates video images with a resolution at almost cellular level, and which can be used for more accurate diagnosis and assessment of macroscopic lesions.

A stool antigen test for *Helicobacter pylori* has been introduced which may represent a useful (considerably cheaper and possibly more convenient) alternative to carbon urea breath tests both for the diagnosis of *H. pylori* infection and to determine the success of eradication therapy.

New drugs for the treatment of irritable bowel syndrome are nearing the market. These are the $5HT_4$-agonists, e.g. tigaserod, and the $5HT_3$-antagonists, of which alosetron is one example. In a recently published trial, alosetron was found to be significantly more effective than mebeverine in women with diarrhoea-predominant IBS. Because IBS is such a common disorder, there is likely to be a significant group of patients who have found previous treatments to be ineffective or who are prompted to consult for the first time when a significantly different new drug is launched. This may have significant cost implications.

Vaccination and chemoprevention

Vaccination against gut pathogens, using predominantly mucosal immunity, is an exciting new development. Live vaccines against *Shigella* and *Salmonella* species are being trialled, and non-living oral vaccines for cholera and enterotoxigenic *E. coli* are available.

Rotavirus is the commonest cause of severe gastroenteritis worldwide. An oral live vaccine has been licensed for use among infants in the USA. The recommended schedule is a three-dose series given at 2, 4 and 6 months of age. The full implementation of this vaccination programme in the USA is expected to prevent most physician visits for rotavirus gastroenteritis and at least two-thirds of hospitalisations and deaths related to rotavirus. Introduction of this vaccine in the UK could have significant effects on the paediatric workload in primary care.

A COX-2 inhibitor has been shown to reduce polyp recurrence in patients at high familial risk of colonic polyps. If this benefit is shown to extend to patients with the much more common sporadic form of polyp, the health economic consequences will be a significant issue for purchasers.

Genetics

The individual patient's risk of colorectal cancer is increased if there is a family history of the disease. The identification of patients whose risk is increased in this way can allow a targeted approach to screening for colorectal cancer, but will require good-quality family history-taking in primary care. Computer programs to enable this are currently under development. These programs will integrate with the existing commercial clinical software packages to operate at the doctor's desk.

Chapter 21

Coding

The importance of accurate and consistent coding

In the world of data management, where terms such as 'electronic health record', 'audit' and 'clinical governance' seem to be mentioned everywhere, accurate coding is essential to ensure that we are all talking the same language. The Read Codes have been a part of all accredited GP systems for some years, but it is often difficult and time-consuming to find the most appropriate code from a myriad of possibilities. The codes which follow have been selected with an understanding of the hierarchical structure as the best if sometimes imperfect fit for the clinical areas that form the body of this publication.

Subject area	Read 5 bit
Dyspepsia (in general, especially when uninvestigated)	J16y4
Gastro-oesophageal reflux disease	J1011
Reflux without oesophagitis	J10y4
Barrett's oesophagitis	J1025
Stricture of oesophagus	J103.
Mallory–Weiss tear	J108.
Achalasia	J100.
Hiatus hernia	J347.
Peptic ulcer disease (unspecified)	J13..
Proven duodenal ulcer	J12..
+ bleeding	J12y1
+ perforation	J12y2
+ both	J12y3
Proven gastric ulcer	J11..
+ bleeding	J11y1
+ perforation	J11y2
+ both	J11y3
Also code if *Helicobacter pylori* is present	A0745
or if induced by non-steroidal	
anti-inflammatory drugs	U6053
Gastritis	J155.
Duodenitis	J157.
Oesophageal cancer	B10..
Gastric cancer	B11..
Haematemesis	J680.
Melaena	J681.
Constipation	J520.
Diarrhoea (functional – no cause found)	J525.
Coeliac disease	J690.
Iron deficiency anaemia	D00..

Gallstones	J64..
Acute cholecystitis	J650.
Choledocholithiasis	J645.
Cholangitis	J661.
Acute pancreatitis	J670.
Chronic pancreatitis	J671.
Viral hepatitis (A, B, C)	A70..
Gastroenteritis	A0812
Irritable bowel syndrome	J521.
Inflammatory bowel disease (unspecified)	J4...
Crohn's disease	J40..
Ulcerative colitis	J4101
Minor anal disorders	
Haemorrhoids	G84..
Fissure	J530.
Fistula in ano	J531.
Pruritus ani	M180.
Perianal warts	A7813
Colorectal cancer	
Caecum	B134.
Ascending colon	B136.
Transverse colon	B131.
Descending colon	B132.
Sigmoid	B133.
Rectum	B141.
Anal canal	B142.

Investigations and diagnostic procedures

Ultrasound examination of the biliary tract	5859.
Barium meal	548..
Barium swallow	547..

Barium enema	54A..
Rigid sigmoidoscopy	771Q
Flexible sigmoidoscopy	771M
Diagnostic proctoscopy	772A
Diagnostic colonoscopy	771J
Oesophageal manometry	780J1
Oesophageal pH monitoring	780J0
Upper gastrointestinal endoscopy	761F
Open cholecystectomy (+ exploration of common bile duct)	78101
Laparoscopic cholecystectomy	78105
Endoscopic retrograde cholangiopancreatography (ERCP) and sphincterotomy	782B.
Extracorporeal shock-wave lithotripsy	78170

Operations to produce stomas should ideally be coded with the exact operation and date. For example:

Hartmann's	77201
Hartmann's – reversal	7729A

Coding systems are continually in a state of flux and new codes are continually being created. The codes themselves are becoming more complicated in an attempt to try to cover more exactly 'all' possible diseases or presentations, but paradoxically they may be simpler to use with fewer 'core' concept codes and a multiple of qualifiers (e.g., left, right, burning, dull, etc.).

The current Read system is being superseded by the combined European/USA Read3/SNOMed coding system within the next few years, but it will be possible for data entered to be automatically 'mapped' to whatever system the future brings, so hours of code-searching will not be wasted!

Index

Indexer: Laurence Errington